A Gradual Disappearance

A Personal Reflection on Living
with Memory Loss

By

ELIZABETH LONSETH

ISBN: 146996550X
ISBN 13: 9781469965505

Dedication and Thanks

To my parents and in-laws who struggled with memory disease.

A special thanks to my husband, Stan Lonseth, for his cover photography and continued support.

Thanks to Brian Grandbouche and Dr. Sameh Elsanadi for their support in the writing of this booklet.

Thank you to my longtime and long-distance friend, Carol Lee Clayton—working together again to stay on the 'same page'!

A portion of the proceeds from the sale of this booklet will be donated to the Alzheimer's Association.

To find out more about Elizabeth Lonseth and her other publications please visit <u>elizabethlonsethnovels.com</u>

Prologues

Dr. Sameh Elsanadi, MD:

Dementia is like a maze. Its victims get lost in the labyrinth of their own minds, bringing confusion and despair to themselves and to others around them. Families watch helplessly as their loved ones drift further and further away from reality, and when decisions are made, emotions often get in the way of what is really necessary. I have spent most of my entire adult life attempting to understand this disease, as well as to provide solace and guidance for afflicted families like Elizabeth's. One of the main steps toward accepting and dealing with this disease, I have found, is to realize that other individuals and families are under the same burden. Elizabeth has provided a great service to the dementia and Alzheimer's community by writing about her family's experience with the disease. Knowledge and information are two of the most helpful tools to aid one in coping with Alzheimer's and dementia, and with the assistance of *A Gradual Disappearance*, managing this disease will become much easier.

Brian Grandbouche, former Executive Director of Aegis of Dana Point:

I have worked in the hospitality, retail, and senior living industries in one way or another for the past thirty years. For the past two years, I have managed a community that specializes in dementia and memory care. One of the greatest gifts I've received while working with seniors is their grace, wisdom, and experience. You learn that at the end of a life well lived, there are only two things that matter most — faith and family. No one is worried about their "stuff" — houses, cars, paintings. The happiest seniors are truly those who have their family around them. When I first heard Elizabeth's idea for *A Gradual Disappearance*, I knew it was perfect. I have had so many conversations with family members and their loved ones, trying to help with the realities of aging and dementia. As I reflect on those conversations, I only wish I could have had this resource to share and help them understand their journey. In this booklet Elizabeth Lonseth shares her personal stories of dealing with loved ones with memory loss disease. She captures how powerful and important your family, friends, and faith are when dealing with the frustration and emotions that go along with taking care of your parents. She gives us page after page of practical advice, wisdom, and grace from someone who has experienced not one, not two, but all four of her parents developing dementia as they grew older. Her insights and personal stories are touching and relatable; it is a must read for anyone coping with a family member with dementia. She will come alongside you as if she were going through it with you, and she has provided a very personal, practical, and powerful book that will help you both emotionally and spiritually and give you hope that you are not alone in this endeavor.

Andrea McDonald, Walk Coordinator, Alzheimer's Association:

Elizabeth, your book tells a true story about a battle that so many people in our community are facing each and every day. The life of a caregiver is better described as the life of an angel. It is through others' experiences that we can learn, and I hope for many in Orange County to learn from your beautiful story, Elizabeth! There are over seventy-five thousand in our community alone affected by, or who are at immediate risk for, Alzheimer's. Your words are here to help. Thank you!

Table of Contents

Notes

Names are not used in this booklet in order to protect individual privacy. Please note the use of both singular and plural pronouns. Reference will be made to male and female patients and at times the singular "they" will be used in an effort to make this booklet more personal to the reader.

The information available about memory disease is being constantly updated as new tests and research projects yield new conclusions. I have tried to provide current and correct information available at the time this booklet was written.

Introduction

M emory disease gradually steals our loved ones away. Silently and subtly it captures them, leaving us wondering where our loved ones went even when they are sitting right in front of us. I hope that sharing what my husband and I have learned as we've walked this difficult path of dementia and Alzheimer's alongside our parents will help others on the same path.

Alzheimer's and dementia are the terms most often used when referring to cognitive impairment. Geriatric psychiatrist Dr. Sameh Elsanadi has explained to me the difference between the two terms as follows:

> **Dementia** is a disease that causes loss of memory and cognitive functions, which impairs the person's ability to function independently. There are several etiologies or causes for dementia.

> **Alzheimer's** is the most common cause of dementia and is simply a degenerative brain disease.

Other types of dementia are vascular dementia, dementia with Lewy bodies, mixed dementia, Parkinson's disease, and frontotemporal lobar degeneration. Definitions and information changes fast as research continues.

My father's dementia during the last two years of his life became an introduction for me. His vascular dementia resulted from fourteen years of heart attacks and strokes, and it gave my husband and I a glimpse of what was to come. At the time I was in my mid-thirties, married for sixteen years, raising three daughters, and busy with a career in interior design. I was not as supportive of my mother as I should have been. I found myself avoiding visiting my parents who lived only an hour and a half away. It was heartbreaking to watch my father, a brilliant forest geneticist, function on the level of a child. Occasionally I would give my mother a break, but I wish now I had done more.

After my father's death, we were given a seven-year respite before my husband and I began the six-year marathon of caring for both of his parents in their home. My father-in-law had Alzheimer's. My mother-in-law had vascular dementia, a result of her many Transient Ischemic Attacks (TIA's) or mini-strokes. Our two older daughters were finished with college and out on their own by the time my in-laws required full-time care. Our youngest daughter was just beginning high school. She helped out after school when she could and on the weekends. When she left for college, we weren't able to enjoy being empty nesters. Instead, my husband and I took turns at his parents' house while struggling to maintain our full-time jobs. During this time writing became a respite for me, which has resulted in two published Christian fiction novels.

As this booklet is being written, we are continuing to deal with my own mother's Alzheimer's. At first I organized caregivers to come into her home; but now she is in a wonderful memory care facility and thoroughly enjoying it.

Humor is a necessity in order to survive this trial. What amazes me is the amount of laughter that occurs in the memory care facility where my mother lives. Often, residents are the ones who make the jokes about their mistakes. Or, if a family member or caregiver tells a joke, the residents love it. Please view the humor in this book with the love and respect I have for my family members. When things got tough, my father always made jokes. My mother used to say, "If we don't laugh, we will cry."

It is essential that we treat the elderly with the respect and dignity they deserve. Illustrating how memory disease destroyed our parents' normal, full, and happy lives is not done with any disrespect for them. My only disdain is for a disease that destroys peoples' minds.

Looking back, there is no single formula or answer to deal with memory disease. Each patient is different and therefore each solution must be an individualized one. However, there are many common threads. I am not a doctor, nor do I have any professional training in this area. All I can offer is the knowledge gained while caring for my parents and my husband's parents. My prayer is that my thoughts and stories will help you.

Elizabeth

Chapter 1

The Unspoken "A" Word — Denial

The ring of the telephone shattered the quietness of the night. My husband jumped out of bed to catch the call. I glanced at the clock. It was two-thirty.

"It's my parents," my husband said, dressing quickly. He dutifully drove the three miles to his parents' house and returned an hour later.

Barely awake, I asked, "What was that about?"

"Slippers," he replied.

"Slippers?" I asked.

"Yeah. My father had taken all my mother's slippers. He wouldn't let her have any of them because he insisted they were his."

My father-in-law, a tailor by trade, took pride in the way he dressed his tall frame. Always sophisticated and appropriate, he was the perfect model for his product. My mother-in-law had elegant and decidedly feminine taste in clothes.

We dozed off to sleep and except for a short discussion in the morning, we forgot about the incident for several years, not recognizing a telltale sign of the Alzheimer's disease that would one day dominate our lives.

Often there are incidents that occur early in the story of an Alzheimer's patient that don't make any sense. These incidents can be isolated, and the senior citizen is able to function normally for a while. However, such incidents should be noted. Loved ones need to be open to the idea that these could be early warning signs of memory disease.

How many times do we hear the phrase, "Oh, he's just getting a little forgetful"? My grandparents' generation called it senility, dismissing any inappropriate behavior with a title. When talking to friends about their parents, I hear this excuse a lot. Yes, we do become forgetful as we age, but odd scenarios could be the early warning signs of much more.

• • •

My mother was one of four sisters. Two passed away from Alzheimer's. One is now over ninety years old, and her mind remains clear. When all four sisters were still living, Alzheimer's became an unspoken word. Forgetful or senile were words they were comfortable with—words that didn't mean out of control or not in one's right mind. The unaffected sisters got upset at their nieces and nephews for stating that their mothers had such a disease. At one point my mother and one of my aunts were considering how to help another sister escape from the facility she had been placed in by her daughter. "She's just a little forgetful, she doesn't need to be in that place," they would say, denying the truth. I could sense the disapproval from my mother when the "A" word was used. Now I realize she was afraid the term might someday be used when speaking of her. She often expressed fear of losing control of her thoughts, but avoiding the word does not prevent its occurrence.

As Mom gradually declined, most of her friends treated her as they always did; greeting her with big smiles and hugs. When attending church with my mother, it was painful to watch two of her oldest friends avoid her. They would look the other direction and walk off as if she had the plague.

• • •

Let's be fair. If a person has always had trouble remembering something it doesn't mean memory issues are the cause. On long walks my husband will often check traffic when we approach a street crossing and tell me the road is clear. I step out into the street without even looking. I trust him with my life. But I do not trust him with my keys. Since the beginning of our marriage almost forty years ago, he has seldom known where his keys are, and has lost a few sets entirely. Losing his keys later in life will not be a sign that he has dementia.

Unfortunately, too many times, signs of memory disease are downplayed. Dementia and Alzheimer's become unspoken words instead of being researched. It is hard to face the fact that your mother or father or even your spouse may have a disease that is destroying their mind and therefore taking him or her away from you. Your parents or spouse need help from someone who is not in denial.

Like a diagnosis of cancer or heart disease, the ramifications of memory disease must not be ignored or the situation will balloon out of control. Preparation and planning make the journey easier. Ignoring it will not make the disease go away. One problem not properly addressed will lead to many more problems. For example, ignoring mobility issues can lead to a fall, resulting in more complicated care. If the doctor told you that your parent had cancer, you would see a specialist, research the type of cancer, and prepare for their medical care. Memory disease needs to be treated in the same way.

Acting normal and hiding moments of forgetfulness is a technique many memory patients employ. Early on in the disease, they can use all their energy to put on a good front for a short period of time. Spend more time with them and you will see their energy wane and telltale signs start to appear such as repeating stories or asking the same questions over and over. Checking in on your parents for an hour once a week will not let you know their mental state.

If you place your loved one in a care facility, friends and acquaintances might think you are misled because they think your parent or spouse is fine. Over twenty years ago, a client of mine asked me to design a studio apartment in a memory care facility for her mother. We met her mother in her condo, and I took inventory of her furniture. I was there for only an hour, and not having much experience yet with the disease, I wondered if my client's mother really needed to live in a memory care facility, she seemed just fine to me. Later on during the installation, I had the privilege of spending time with the sweet, delightful mother. After the first hour had passed, it became very apparent why she needed memory care. She could put on a front for awhile, but then her true mental state surfaced.

• • •

The inability to learn new tasks is an indication of Alzheimer's. My mother has always been a major organizer. President of two garden clubs and the weavers' guild, as well as a Bible Study Fellowship leader, planning was her forte. One year we made the mistake of upgrading her iMac computer to a newer model with a slightly different file organizing system. My husband spent three different long afternoons carefully showing her all the new commands and I spent an hour or two every week helping her, but she never mastered the system. In fact, I often heard her tell her friends, "No one has bothered to teach me how to use it." When you start to get frustrated with your parent repeatedly about the same issue, it's time to ask why.

Sometimes it's not a new task but an old task that the patient can no longer perform. They simply cannot follow through with it, no matter how many times they are reminded or explanations are given.

At first my husband and I were just helping with the daily chores at my in-laws' home — the bills, grocery shopping, etc. We were each in the house at least once a day and we started to notice that the house always seemed to be at either subzero or sauna temperatures. My father-in-law had begun to play with the thermostat. My husband reminded him repeatedly not to touch the heat, but it didn't help. Finally we put a lockable clear plastic cover over the thermostat so only we could adjust it. Years later, when we cleaned out my father-in-law's desk, we found a notebook filled with one sentence, repeated line after line, page after page, in his handwriting; "Do not touch the heat." It is hard to accept the fact that those we love won't be getting better. Even though they might act like two-year-olds they aren't and sadly, they can't learn and grow like children can.

Besides being an organizer, my mom liked being in charge. I could care less about a lot of things so that is one reason our mother-daughter relationship was a good one. She enjoyed doing the planning and the driving. Mom dreamed of vacationing in Hawaii. She had been through the Honolulu airport on the way to other destinations but had never visited the beaches and the sights on Oahu. In the spring of 2005, she got a deal through her credit card, and by splitting the costs we could afford the trip. Mom handed me the brochure and said, "You book it." I should have known then that something was wrong.

A month after we booked the trip, my mother-in-law passed away. Then, in the fall, two weeks before our trip, my father-in-law also went to be with the Lord. I immediately planned to cancel the trip, but my husband insisted I still go with my mother to Hawaii.

Mom and I made a list of things she wanted to do on the island. Although I tried several times before we left to plan an itinerary with her, she was always too busy. I decided to leave that task for the five-hour plane ride.

While waiting to board, my mother asked who would be driving the rental car.

"Aren't you?" I asked, surprised she had even brought up the subject.

"Why don't you drive?" she suggested.

On the plane I again tried to get her input on which days we should do what, but she evaded my questions and slept for four hours instead. I spent the plane trip trying to memorize the roads and layout of Oahu, realizing I would not have a navigator to help me.

During our first evening at the resort, several attempts to engage my mother in the planning process failed. The next morning I knew I had to make the decisions myself and move on. All of this bothered me a bit, but I didn't dwell on it. I was determined to make it a dream vacation for her.

I had looked forward to hours on the beach or by the pool having long, deep conversations with Mom. That never happened. She became obsessed with the children playing nearby and often ignored me completely. The fourth day at our resort, she got lost on the way back up to our room; a task she had been completing successfully by herself for three days.

Going to dinner each night became difficult. The lady that could once out-hike anyone else in the woods could now barely walk. She blamed her dress shoes for not fitting right. After the first night, I purchased shoe pads to help. She still shuffled her way to dinner in the tiniest baby steps. At times she even had trouble with her walking shoes.

Upon our return home, I scheduled a doctor's appointment for the following week, hoping the doctor would be able to offer an explanation for Mom's strange behavior. Mom showed up for the appointment bright and perky, able to perform every physical and mental task the doctor required. The doctor gave me the "you are crazy" look and let me know there was nothing wrong with my mother.

Later on, I learned that plane travel can disorient memory patients. The long ride had confused Mom enough to give me a glimpse of the future. Unlike the typical pattern of Alzheimer's, in which the mental skills go first and then the physical, Mom's motor skills declined first. She has now been wheelchair-bound for over a year.

At Christmas of 2005, we noticed more warning signs that my mother had Alzheimer's. The smell of turkey roasting in the oven greeted us at the front door, but once in the kitchen it became evident that nothing else had been prepared. Mom looked at me, walked into the living room, sat down in her chair, and announced, "I am going to enjoy Christmas this year." My sister-in-law and I looked at each other in shock. Was Mom abandoning her kitchen? Without even asking if we wanted to help? We put on aprons and, with the help of our daughters, prepared, served, and cleaned up after the meal.

I reacted in anger. It had only been four months since my father-in-law had passed away, and I realized we would be traveling down the same road again, with my mother. Thankfully, several months later the Lord gave me peace with the thought, "She is in no pain."

• • •

If your loved one has memory issues, your experiences will naturally differ from ours in specific ways, but there will be general similarities. Each brain is affected in a distinct way. The self-defense mechanism of denial wants to gloss over the problems and ignore them. Try to be as objective as you can for the sake of your spouse or parent, and for your own sake. Objectivity will help you find the appropriate care for your loved one and at the right time.

Chapter 2

Sundowners, Strange Behavior, and Acting Out

I walked through the back door of my in-law's home and into the kitchen, knowing that my daughter had left fifteen minutes earlier. She had called informing me that both of my in-laws were in their chairs napping. That usually meant that I would have to wake them up, but not today. There at the counter stood my father-in-law with his largest kitchen knife, chopping onions. I could tell he was already on his second onion by the size of the pile on the plate in front of the chopping board.

"How are you?" I asked.

He grunted in reply instead of offering his usual cheery, "Hi."

"What are you doing?" I asked.

He gave me a dumbfounded look. "Chopping onions for dinner."

I suggested that maybe he had chopped enough.

He lips tightened, and he raised his voice. "Mom says she needs three chopped onions for dinner."

Since "Mom" referred to his own mother, who had died thirty-five years before, I decided it was best to drop the subject. I moved into the living room and woke up my mother-in-law to take her to the bathroom, wondering who forgot to put the knife away. By the time we returned to the living room, my father-in-law was sitting in his chair, smiling and glad to see me. In the kitchen, I rinsed the knife and put it away in the pantry, which we kept locked.

Another symptom of dementia is sundowning. Wikipedia explains, "A person who is sundowning may exhibit mood swings, become abnormally demanding, suspicious, upset or disoriented, and see or hear things that are not there in the late afternoon or evening."[1] Sundown syndrome usually manifests itself in the late afternoon or early evening in some kind of repetitive agitated behavior.

Dr. Elsanadi believes that sundowners "act out because of the build-up of frustration, tiredness, nervousness, and discomfort of being a dementia patient who can't communicate their needs over the course of a day." He adds, "It is almost like having a period of transient delirium in the late-afternoon or early evening time due to a dis-regulation of the cholinergic system in the brain." Elsanadi also maintains that "the agitation is a form of anxiety that is tied to disruption of the biological clocks of older people with dementia where their sleep-wake cycles are fragmented. This fragmentation causes further escalation of the chemical imbalances which could make the person aggressive, restless, and delusional."[2]

My mother in-law used to pace inside the house for half an hour straight, making a circle from the living room, through the hall and other rooms arriving back at her chair, sitting for two minutes, and starting all over again. The activity helped keep her mobile and eased her restlessness, but it was annoying at times.

My father-in-law wore a three-inch deep hole in the upholstered arm of his favorite chair by rubbing and clawing at it with his fingers. We had to retire the chair when he began to eat the exposed foam.

When she still lived in her own home, my mother used to see imaginary gangs of men on the road up the hill. The trees and bushes had grown so that the road could no longer be seen from the house. She asked us if we saw the men, and if we said no, she became agitated.

Sundowning can occur at other times in the day, as well. One night my daughter, who was then living with my mother, woke to loud noises in Grandma's room. She found her grandma packing suitcases full of clothes, photos, and files from her desk drawer. Her room was a mess. When my daughter questioned her, Mom had no idea where she was going. It took several hours for my daughter to convince her to give up the project and go to sleep.

• • •

Another strange behavior in memory patients can be weird eating habits — like eating a pound of butter or a whole loaf of bread at one sitting. We had to hide food from my father-in-law because he didn't know when to stop eating. I have heard of families that have caught their loved one trying to eat dirt in the backyard. Like toddlers, dementia patients no longer know what is good for them and what is not. They often wander, not knowing where they're going or rummage through things, not sure of what they're looking for.

Often dementia patients live in a world of unreality. My mother currently exists in her early twenties. One of the residents asked her on her last birthday if she was twenty-five yet.

Mom gave her an incredulous look and announced with a giggle, "I hope I'm not that old!"

Seeing the humor in her pronouncement, I asked, "How do you explain me? I'm fifty-nine." Everyone, including my mother, laughed.

My in-laws' neighbors in Seattle once contacted us to express concern because my father-in-law kept offering to take them to lunch in his hometown of Molde, Norway. He firmly believed that if they drove over the Ballard Bridge near his home and turned right, they would be in Molde. Trying to explain to him that he was living in another country became a futile effort. Correcting memory patients doesn't work and often leads to frustration. We decided to agree with my father-in-law and drop the subject.

The disease can also change personalities. A proud, stubborn, my-way-or-no-way personality like my father-in-law's can become docile and grateful for the smallest help as the disease progresses. Unfortunately, the reverse is also true; the sweetest little lady can become grouchy and mean-spirited and start acting out.

Alzheimer's often goes through stages, as it gradually destroys memory, reason, judgment, speech, and motor skills. It is unfortunately impossible to predict which area will be affected in each individual or to what degree.

• • •

Besides dealing with your loved one's care, you will also have to deal with your own emotions. Anger, hurt, confusion, or despair may surprise you, but they are normal reactions. Anger can hit when you take on a task that they used to do.

You think, "I shouldn't have to do this. Why didn't they clean out this garage or the basement years ago?"

It is painful to watch and hard to understand as your wonderful parent or spouse turns into someone you don't recognize, someone who is sometimes out of control and possibly violent. It is difficult because these loved ones often act like small children, yet we can't pick them up and put them in time out. We have to consider their own safety and the safety of others. Often they refuse help, not wanting anyone to invade the privacy of their home. Working with them can be trying. It is important to consult professional advice, so behavior issues can be properly addressed.

Chapter 3

Coming Alongside

How do you deal with the ramifications of memory loss? At first my husband and I made the mistake of trying to correct his parents' behavior and attempted to help them learn again what they had lost. That didn't work. They only became frustrated and more agitated. We began to try to figure out where they were in their head at the moment — maybe sixteen again, or in another part of the world. My cousin told me to ask them "How old are you today?" Their answers often gave us clues as to how to interact with them.

Our parents taught us not to lie. Well, now is the time to break that rule. Agreements and even promises that you know you won't keep go a long way in keeping things stable. Dementia patients quickly forget the promises and agreeing with them can calm them down. Maybe it isn't really lying, but simply entering the reality that they're living in. When your parent thinks you are a brother or sister, play along. Keeping everyone calm and happy is the goal.

Distraction is another great tool when caring for dementia patients. Get them involved in a project, play a game, have a snack, or take a little walk inside or outside. Activities keep their deteriorating minds occupied and in the present.

Humor helps. Make jokes about yourself or tell a joke. Keeping an upbeat, happy atmosphere seems to diffuse some of the antagonism often manifested by the memory-impaired and it will also help your attitude and give you peace of mind.

Learning to put things on the back burner is another successful technique. When my in-laws' house needed a new roof, my husband, who is an architect, got a bid from a roofer he had used many times in the past. He presented the estimate of roughly five thousand dollars to his father. His father said no, that he had to find someone who could do it for a thousand dollars and no more. Knowing this was impossible; my husband took a closer look at the roof and determined it would last another winter. The next fall the same roofer returned and, for a slightly higher price, put a new roof on the house. My father-in-law sat inside for two days, happily watching TV, unaware that four men were walking around his yard and pounding away on the roof above his head. As the disease progresses, some things do get easier as the patients let go, allowing you to take over tasks entirely.

When talking to a caregiver or a doctor, try not to talk about the patient when the patient is present. Instead, include your loved one in the conversation. When a caregiver is trying to figure out your mother's eating patterns, ask your mother, "Well, you like to eat early, right, Mom?" I can always sense my mother slumping and trying to disappear when someone talks about her as if she isn't in the room. Memory patients sense what is going on, and it affects them. Ignoring their presence could become a catalyst for aggressive behavior.

Memory patients often know they are losing control. It wears them down to be told what to do all day long. They feel useless and may become angry, which can lead to shutting down or acting out. It is important that we try to refrain from directing them; instead, we should give them options and let them make a few decisions. Who cares if their socks don't match their pants for one day? Giving them back some control will make them happier.

Why placate the memory-impaired? If you don't, they can spiral into aggressive behavior. When we don't come alongside by entering our loved one's reality they can become momentarily aware of their mental limitations resulting in acting out — hitting, biting, or even attacking others. They can become physically stronger during these outbursts.

Learning to let go and accept our loved one's mental capacity as it is can be tough. Don't try to change them, however; learn to join them. This doesn't apply to destructive behavior, of course. When your mother imagines she is in her early twenties and dating again, let it go. Listen to her ramblings, agree when she notices a handsome young man, and move on to another subject. Acceptance is the key, not reorientation.

Chapter 4

Finding the Appropriate Care

How do you find the right care for your loved one? A visit to the doctor is a good place to start. Though at this time, there is no specific medical test for Alzheimer's per se, a comprehensive evaluation, which includes cognitive and laboratory tests can assist the physician in giving you a diagnosis. By conducting the laboratory tests first, the doctor may find medical conditions which display Alzheimer's-like symptoms. Laboratory tests may detect a treatable condition like depression, medication side effects, thyroid problems, or low vitamin B12. All these can contribute to mental disorientation. Once the treatable conditions are ruled out the doctor may require a MRI, PET scans and possibly an EEG to distinguish between Alzheimer's, seizures, or strokes. When the doctor knows all other possible diseases and conditions are not the cause of your loved one's confusion, Alzheimer's is a possibility. The cognitive test of your loved one's functional ability gives further confirmation and will help you in determining the appropriate level of care.

You should be involved with all doctor appointments because your parent or spouse will not accurately remember what the doctor said. Even worse, they could become confused about prescribed medication. Developing a good working relationship with the doctor is valuable. The physician can be the "bad guy" and inform your parent they can no longer drive or that they need help in a certain area. My mother loved Dr. L., but once Dr. L. suggested that Mom stop driving, Mom complained about her for many months, declaring her a traitor.

One trick I learned was to stand or sit behind my mother-in-law where she couldn't see me. I let her answer the questions the doctor asked, but I was able to shake my head yes or no and give signals to the doctor as to the truth of her answers. This gave the doctor an idea of her mental capacity. From my position of invisibility, I often was amazed to hear my mother-in-law's (and now my mother's) irrational view of life. Many doctors will also want to meet with you privately so that you can talk freely about your parent or spouse.

• • •

So your parent or spouse has been diagnosed with dementia or Alzheimer's. What do you do now? If it is possible, discuss care options with your loved one, making your loved one part of the process. This may not work with patients who refuse to face the facts and act out when presented with them.

How do we know what type of care is right? Should we keep our loved ones in their homes? Should we relocate them to care facilities? Just as this disease affects each person in a unique way, there is a unique answer for each one's care.

The Internet is a helpful tool when making decisions about care. Use a search engine to find local agencies that could be helpful during this time. Many cities and counties post lists on their websites of organizations that can help. You are your loved one's advocate, so be careful to choose reputable organizations. Consider contacting the local Alzheimer's Association. Catholic Community Services provides care services for Catholics and non-Catholics alike.

A helpful website I've found is www.aplaceformom.com. This website provides assistance at no charge to find affordable care for seniors. Consider using the National Council on Aging website at www.ncoa.com. Through the NCOA you can obtain information on ombudsman services, socialization/mental health programs, the Friendly Visitor Program, the Financial Abuse Specialist Team, and the Medicare Fraud Unit.

There are many different types of care to consider. If you decide residing at home is the best for your loved one, there are in-home caregivers — both private individuals and agencies. Research these agencies, because even if you want to take care of your loved yourself, you will need a break or additional help at times.

There are adult family homes where a family cares for two to four patients in their home. The family lives in one area of the home and the patients in another. There are adult family homes that are fully staffed by professional caregivers where the patients are the only residents.

Senior living facilities range from home-like to mega villages in size. These facilities offer independent living, assisted living, or memory care. Some senior living facilities provide all three levels of care, allowing the resident to stay in the same place throughout their decline and end of life. Usually senior living facilities require a non-refundable deposit in addition to the monthly rent. These facilities also vary by the type of care they provide, the quality, and the price. For those patients who remain in their own home, there is respite care available through senior living facilities, which will care for patients for a week or two to give their caregivers a break.

Proper placement for your loved one depends on his or her functional ability. This is one of the reasons having a reputable doctor familiar with dementia is crucial; a doctor's assessment will help you find the right living situation for your parent(s).

At the end of this journey, you might need the services of hospice. It is not a government-run program. Hospice care comes from private companies that are operating for profit, and a doctor must initiate the order for hospice. It can be provided in a caring, supportive way, but some of it may be poorly run. Because many memory patients are in need of this service, it is important to understand that you have a choice. You can change companies if you need to. We found that going through hospice at the end of life can make the legal aspects easier. You will have fewer questions to answer as the coroner and police will have access to necessary information, which will speed up the cause of death inquiry.

• • •

I hope the following personal illustrations about caring for my parents gives you more insight in selecting the type of care for your loved one.

My father was still in the early stages of dementia when he passed away so my mother was able to help him with his simple needs by providing his meals, helping him button his shirts, and managing his medications. He could still carry on a conversation, bathe and dress himself, and take care of his toileting needs. He remained well oriented at home but sometimes became confused when they were away from home.

My in-laws made my husband promise that they would die in their home. We kept that promise, but due to falls or illnesses, they were each hospitalized twice and subsequently placed temporarily in a skilled nursing facility or in an adult family home to convalesce. During these instances they acted out, resulting in my husband almost living at those facilities. Once they returned home, they calmed down and went back to their daily routines. Though not ideal, their bathroom met their handicapped needs, because they stayed relatively mobile until the end. We brought in occasional, temporary in-home care when we needed a break. These caregivers came to us from reputable agencies. Our three grown daughters each helped out at various times. The last four months of my father-in-law's life, however, we needed extra help on a regular basis.

Caring for a parent or parents in their own homes can be stressful, time-consuming and at times, inconvenient. Because this method of care does not have built-in support from a team of caregivers, in-home care by family members can become a vortex that pulls you in gradually and swallows you up, if it is not well planned. When you are in the middle of a tornado, it's too late to build a storm cellar. Home care by family members should be planned out carefully. Foresight for possible future situations resulting from expected or unexpected changes should be part of any planning process.

My mother designed herself out of her house. When she remodeled thirty years before her illness, she rejected my husband's design for a spacious master bath. Once that side of the house was demolished and she could visualize the possibilities, she decided a private bath might be nice after all, but instead of using my husband's design, she sketched up a bathroom that would make airline interior designers jealous. Neither of the two remaining bathrooms provided enough space for someone to assist her. So, as her mobility decreased and her assistance needs increased, it became apparent she could no longer stay at home.

Information about Americans with Disabilities Act (ADA) regulations is available online at www.ADABathroom.com. These regulations provide grab bar heights, the space required for using a wheelchair or walker, and other valuable information for ease of function. Remodeling a bathroom might make it possible for the patient to remain at home longer.

I organized private in-home care for my mother at first. Through Mom's church we located a private caregiver who ended up being a gift from the Lord. She worked twenty to thirty hours a week, mornings through mid-afternoon. At first Mom would microwave her own dinner, but when she lost that skill, a neighbor girl was hired to put Mom's dinner in the microwave and chat with her while she ate. She and Mom became quite close. As we needed more help, a friend of my daughter's who was attending nursing school became the afternoon/evening caregiver. Sometimes she brought in dinner and she, her husband, and daughter would join Mom for a nice family meal. Occasionally she would take Mom to church and back to her own house for Sunday lunch. Two of my daughters took turns living with their grandma so the night shift and weekends were covered. I came in every Thursday to give everyone a break and take Mom to the hairdresser, to grocery shop, and to get medications. Many times this involved a Wednesday night flight from my new home in California. (That got old really fast.) I was running an adult family home for one. I survived on lists and created schedules for meals and caregivers on the plane. Group emails with the month's schedule turned out to be a lifesaver.

Now my mother lives in a memory care facility a mile from our house and I enjoy visiting her every day when I'm not traveling for business. Since I am no longer her caregiver and running a memory care center for one in her own house, I have returned to spending leisure time with her. Instead of calling me her sister or mother, she introduces me as her daughter again. Sometimes my visits are short, other times we sit and talk out in the gardens, put puzzles together, and visit nearby parks to view the ocean. She enjoys Bible study, book club, exercise sessions, chair volleyball, ball toss, and singing, all provided on her level.

• • •

For us, each method of care we chose worked at a particular time. You will have to evaluate and decide which type of care is right for your loved one. Before deciding on in-home care by family members and/or yourself, carefully consider the stress it will place on the one or ones providing the care. Hiring in-home care will require interviews and checking of references. If an adult care home or senior living is the choice, visit several facilities keep your eyes open for problems. Check with your local ombudsman to see if there have been any complaints about any potential facility. There are places and people that do not provide good care. You have to be hands-on, dropping in and checking on the situation.

Try to stay objective when evaluating a loved one's needs so that you can select the proper care, especially if you have chosen a care facility. I have observed many memory patients move into the facility where my mother lives. I have seen cases where the family members insist their loved one must be placed in assisted care. The new resident has difficulty adjusting to their new home and after several more assessments, it is determined that the best situation for them is to be moved to a memory care unit. The resident feels more at home in the memory care unit, receives crucial one-on-one attention, and begins to thrive. Remember memory patients' needs change often, and sometimes rapidly. Maintain a close watch. Plan ahead for the next phase to help alleviate stress.

Finances will play a part in your decision for care. If a patient's home is paid for, it is cheaper to keep the patient there until the patient's physical needs require full-time care. If funds are limited, do some research to find agencies that can help with in-home care. Check with the Veterans Administration if your loved one served in the military. There might be available benefits. Many communities have agencies that prepare and deliver meals for a low cost to those who qualify as lower income.

• • •

Spousal care has to be the hardest type of care. The emotions and ties are closer than with parents because of the romantic love shared over the years. A spouse is a life partner and best friend. Maybe you promised yourself you'd take care of your spouse at home. If you let anyone else in as a caregiver, or move your spouse to a care facility, you may feel guilty or believe you have failed. This is far from the truth. Just as certain physical conditions require skilled nursing at some point, memory disease may require professional care. Do not hibernate in your home; reach out for help. Try to stay objective enough to make the right decisions. Spouses often will sacrifice their own health while caring for a partner and the stress can bring on heart attacks, strokes, or other health concerns. If you die first, who will take care of your spouse?

Do you have siblings or other family members who are willing to help? Develop a plan to share the duties between those willing and able to help. Take turns helping or visiting. What about resources available from the patient's church? Is there a program in place for visiting the elderly? Some community centers offer adult day care; if mobility isn't a problem, this may be a solution for a time.

Chapter 5

Finances

One of the first signs of memory disease is often an inability to understand finances. Every month my father-in-law called my husband about a certain bill he owed and asked him to come over to help him pay it. By the time my husband arrived at their house, my father-in-law would have forgotten about the bill. They searched his desk without success. Finally, after six months, my husband found the bill. It was from Macy's, but there was an eight-hundred-dollar credit on the account. My father-in-law had been paying the same amount each month not realizing he owed nothing.

If you do not already have both a medical and financial power of attorney (POA) in place, make sure to obtain them. You will need them while dealing with banks, hospitals and other institutions, like the Social Security Administration. Go to each of the financial institutions your loved one does business with and get your name on all the accounts. If possible, set a limit on the amount the patient can withdraw.

My father-in-law once closed a large savings account and withdrew all the money in a cashier's check. It took us several weeks to locate the check he had hidden in the house. That alone was a nuisance, but this account also happened to be the account that his Norwegian pension was deposited into each month. It took my husband three months of working with the Norwegian pension agency to get his father's benefit reinstated with a new bank account, one that his father could not close.

If we can become involved with our senior citizen's finances early, while they are still mentally sound, they will be able to pass along helpful information. Going over the mail together is a good way to ease into private affairs. Junk mail becomes very confusing for memory patients; what could be a scam may look like a bill to their confused minds. Set up a time to go over bills and income together each month. This will require maximum patience on your part since you could pay all the bills in half the time it will take to review one bill with a memory patient. But writing a check for a utility bill may remind your loved one of a bank account they keep for paying the household bills. An account you knew nothing about. Suspicion makes some people resist letting others see their finances. Gradually gain their trust. If all else fails enlist another family member to take the patient on an outing while you go through the desk. It is best to have a good working knowledge of household affairs so that payments aren't missed, stocks sold at a loss, or senior discounts (such as property taxes) aren't forfeited. Some counties allow for senior discounts or exemptions for elderly property taxes. You don't want to lose this "earned" privilege.

Dementia patients usually phase themselves out of finances as their minds are no longer able to deal with it. You will then be free to use your own system of keeping track of the finances. Many seniors use slower, more out-of-date methods, and you may have to take some time to improve things. I have found it helpful to create computer spreadsheets for financial, medical, and personal affairs. I also found it helpful to keep separate notebooks of financial, medical, and social (Christmas card list, church items, organizations, etc.) matters. Having a financial contact sheet that lists each business or institution we dealt with, the contact person at each, contact info, and date when I sent Mom's power of attorney to the business, has saved me time. Many times a customer service representative would say, "We have no record of a power of attorney on file, and we cannot discuss the details of your parent's account with you." Being able to state the date I sent the power of attorney sped things up. Most businesses or financial institutions are helpful, while others may treat you like you are an enemy.

Becoming involved early with your loved one's finances will save you time in the long run. I wish I had taken over my mother's checkbook sooner; when I finally did it took me over two months to unravel the mess and figure out what she had been up to.

Checkbooks, credit cards, and cash will need to be supervised. At one of my recent book signings, an elderly lady walked up, opened her checkbook and offered to buy all the books on my table. I thanked her politely but declined. As we talked, it became apparent to me that she was suffering from some kind of dementia. She became insistent that she wanted to buy a book, so I gave in and signed a copy for her then spent several minutes helping her fill out the check. When she left, I shook my head, thinking that if I had been dishonest, I could have had the best book-signing ever and filled in any amount on the check I wanted. Instead, I contacted another lady who knew the family, asked her to alert the family about the situation, and offered to return the check for the book if the family so desired.

Taking away financial privileges should be a gradual transition. Start by asking questions about your loved one's day and inquiring about how things were paid for. Make it a normal part of everyday conversation. Don't come across as bossy or controlling, because that will quickly shut down communication. Ease in slowly.

So now I have told you to snoop, another thing our parents always taught us not to do. As they lose the ability to care for themselves, our parents lose their privacy, and it's better that they lose it to their children than to someone else. There may be other rules you'll find yourself breaking.

Chapter 6

Driving

Recently at an Alzheimer's driving seminar, Dr. Joanne Marie Hamilton stated that "the difference between an Alzheimer's patient and a dementia patient is that the dementia patient is aware of the loss of driving ability while the Alzheimer's patient has delusions of being a good driver." [3]

Her statement reminded me of when my father-in-law's driver's license was due for renewal, my husband didn't tell him about it but just let it expire. Whenever he was asked by someone if he had a driver's license, my father-in-law would reply, "I don't need a license. The DMV sent me a letter telling me I am such a good driver I don't need a license." He naturally could never find the letter if asked to prove it.

At the seminar I also learned that our driving skills start to diminish in our forties, and our response time lengthens because the brain is less flexible. Most types of dementia affect attention span, which can be dangerous on the road. In rare cases the memory patient can forget which pedal is the gas and which is the brake.

Dr. Joanne Hamilton explained, "A 75 to 84-year-old driver is equivalent to a teenager on the road. Instead of being overly aggressive, the elderly are hyper-careful, making them just as dangerous. Unable to jump from one stimulus to another, they become easily distracted and their visual organization is impaired."[3]

Car trips can disorient some elderly drivers. My father often forgot where he was going toward the end of his life, but he fortunately returned home safely the few times he managed to get the keys. On one trip across the state of Washington, my mother, who was riding in the middle seat of our van, firmly believed we were on an airplane.

Memory patients can put on a good front for a short period of time and fool you into thinking they are still alert enough to drive. Take a ride with your parent on a regular basis to assess their skills. Double-check all medications to make sure none of the medications impair driving skills, or conflict with other medications your loved one is taking.

Removing your parents' driving privileges removes their freedom. It also means more work for you, since you must then provide for their transportation needs. It is better to deal with this inconvenience than to deal with a lawsuit over damaged property or worse, someone else's death.

It can be difficult to take away driving privileges from a person with Alzheimer's who cannot recognize his or her diminished skills. If discussion of giving up driving privileges causes agitation for your loved one, try a gradual approach — arrange for rides and for groceries to be delivered, slowly phasing out the patient's need to drive. Some communities provide elder vans that for a small fee take seniors to the doctor, the shopping mall, or wherever else they need to go. If possible, quietly take the keys out of the house when the patient isn't aware of it. The diminished ability to function may eventually keep a patient from wanting to drive at all; it becomes too much work as energy levels decline.

As mentioned before, use a doctor's instructions as a reason to take away the keys. It is also a good idea to research state laws about senior drivers. Some states require the elderly to renew their licenses with increased frequency, and to renew in person instead of mailing in a renewal application. A few states require retesting at a certain age. Other states require doctors to report certain physical ailments.

Chapter 7

Medications, Vision, Dental, and Hearing Needs

A t some point you will need to take over the dispensing of your loved one's medications. When we had to do this for my mother-in-law, we initially thought we could accomplish it by purchasing a weekly pillbox with a place for pills to be taken each day of the week and at each meal. It worked for a week or two, then pills started to disappear before the scheduled day, and we realized we had to lock the medication away and dispense it ourselves. Confusion, illness, or even death can be caused by improper consumption of prescription or over-the-counter drugs.

It is important to know the medications your loved one is taking and any potential side effects. A doctor may prescribe one of several medications that help slow down the progression of Alzheimer's. I know of cases where these have seemed to help, and the patient is not affected by possible side effects.

Both my father-in-law and my mother could not tolerate the medication and suffered from severe indigestion and aggravation as a result.

I found it helpful to create a spreadsheet that lists all medications, including dosage and frequency of consumption, plus the pharmacy and doctor phone numbers for renewal and usage questions. Such a list is helpful for caregivers in your home and you will need it to move into any senior living facility.

If your loved one acts out to the point of being dangerous to themselves or others, there are medications that may help. In the care of our parents, my husband and I were fortunate to be able to avoid those for the most part. The doctor prescribed a low dosage for my father-in-law's sundowners and it was enough to take the edge off and keep him functional. There are specialists like Dr. Elsanadi, a board-certified geriatric psychiatrist, who can determine which medication may help treat that kind of behavior. Through proper care, this behavior can be modified and patients can return to a calmer life. Discuss any possible side effects with the doctor.

Having medications mailed can be a positive or a negative thing. A dementia patient should not receive medications when no one else is present. Mailing can save you time, but make sure a responsible person receives or signs for the delivered package.

Giving medication to memory patients can become a problem. They may become paranoid, thinking you are trying to make them sick or poison them. Take time to explain the pills and what each one is for in simple, nonthreatening terms.

If possible, attend appointments for vision, dental, and hearing check-ups while your loved one can still respond properly to the doctor or dentist. This will help you learn details that you will need to know in the future. As our loved ones' mental and communication abilities diminish, taking care of these needs becomes harder.

My mother-in-law was hard of hearing. In the early stages of her dementia, she was able to tell her doctor what worked or didn't work when she needed a new hearing aid. As the years passed, she could no longer communicate or even recognize when the battery went dead, so we began to change the batteries on a regular basis.

My mother now believes she can see fine with or without her glasses, although it is evident that is not true.

Mobility can become an issue for appointments. If you decide to place your loved one in a memory care facility, be sure to find out if the facility has doctors, dentists and vision care providers who come in regularly to attend to patients' needs.

Chapter 8

Making Time for Yourself: Don't feel guilty for taking a break

Respite for family members and caregivers is a necessity, an absolute necessity. The unreality in which your loved one lives can be exhausting and the disease in general can be harder on the families than the person suffering from it. Even when you've had a good night's rest, when dealing with the consequences of this disease your own life can cease to make sense and it is easy to become ensnared in a tunnel of unreality. You are constantly under physical, mental, and emotional stress, whether you realize it or not. You are mourning your loved ones while they are still alive, which is exhausting. You need to take time away from the situation.

Simple changes in your parent's needs or living situation can also wear you down. Just moving them from a single room to a shared room in a care facility can take a toll on you. When my mother moved from a private room to one shared with a roommate I cried. It seemed silly to cry over something that simple, but moving her furniture forced me to face her diminishing abilities which hit me hard.

Taking a break can give you a more objective view when you return and help you make better decisions for your loved one. When I return from a long business trip, it is amazing the clearer perspective I have of Mom's situation. If providing in-home care, even an hour break can make a difference in your mental state. Change your normal routine. Do something that recharges you. Take a day trip or go to the movies. Reward yourself with your favorite pastime such as reading, walking, shopping, bike riding, or swimming.

However, getting away for several days or even a week is the best. Rest and relax to prevent your own collapse; your loved ones depend on you to stay healthy for them.

Find a support group in your area and make time to attend at least once a month. It helps to know there are others out there going through the same thing. Another member may offer a suggestion that helps you, or you may have the privilege of helping others.

Are there friends or relatives who could come once a month or once a week to visit your loved one or take on a few duties to give you a break? Make caring for your loved one more of a team effort. Let this experience be one that brings the family together, not one that tears it apart.

Keep up your own health. Don't neglect doctor and dentist appointments. Tell your doctor you are a caregiver; your physician will understand the amount of stress you are under and can watch for signs that stress is taking a toll on your health. Work out regularly and eat right. Stay strong for your loved one. In a normal state of mind, your loved one would want you to take care of yourself. Don't give into guilt when you take a break. It is a necessity.

Keep a balance in your life. I have watched family members destroy relationships by sacrificing their own life to take care of parents or a spouse. I have also seen people drop their parent off at a facility and seldom visit them. I cannot judge, as I do not know the situation. However we do have a responsibility to make sure loved ones are properly cared for.

Find humor in situations and dwell on the good moments with your loved one. Mentally record the times you hear "I love you," or when eyes light up when you walk in the room. Out of the blue my mother recently said "Thank you for all you have done for me. Thank you for taking care of me." Then she returned to her unreality, prattling on, not finishing sentences, nor making any sense.

At times you may wonder if you are suffering from memory disease. Listen to these feelings and take a break.

I knew things had to change when the "great peanut butter incident of 2009" occurred. As I alluded to earlier, in 2008 and 2009, we had a crazy schedule. A typical week started out on Friday night or Sunday night leaving our boat and flying out of Seattle to our home in California. My husband would work Monday through Wednesday in California overseeing an architectural project. We flew back to Seattle on Wednesday night so that he could be in the Seattle office Thursday morning. Early Thursday morning I would drive an hour and a half to Mom's and take over for the caregivers. Mom and I did errands in town and I would shop for groceries while she was at the hairdressers. Each week I drove three different cars, as Mom could not get in or out of my vehicle. Every week I would also shop at three different grocery stores for three different households. Sometimes I would pause in the grocery aisle and remind myself where I was and *who* I was shopping for. With the use of extensive lists that I compiled while on the plane, things seemed to be under control until we needed peanut butter. For three weeks in a row I bought peanut butter. At the end of those three weeks, Mom had three and a half jars but our California home and our boat in Seattle didn't have any. I knew one of the places needed peanut butter but I could not remember which one. I even asked my doctor if I had early-onset Alzheimer's. She assured me it was the result of my hectic life.

• • •

A humorous incident may help keep you going. Enjoy those moments. For most of the thirty-five years we lived in Seattle, my husband and I always shopped at the same grocery store. We knew all the clerks by name and could zip through picking up a week's worth of groceries in twenty minutes. His parents shopped at another local food market. When he first started getting groceries for his parents they insisted he shop at their store.

Several years into caring for his parents my husband left to help them get ready for bed. After he left, I decided I could use the time to get the groceries done. I was sailing through the store with a full cart, trying to be considerate of the few other shoppers. Rounding the corner, I hit another cart head on. It was my husband, shopping for his parents. He had decided to stop shopping at his parents' store and start shopping at our store. After we got over our surprise we laughed and continued shopping. That night it became a game, each of us trying to beat the other to the checkout stands. I forget who made it first, but we both enjoyed the clerks' double takes when they saw each of us with full carts.

The clerk checking me out cleared his throat and ventured to ask, "Did you know that your husband is two aisles over with a full cart?"

"Yes," I replied.

"Are you two okay?"

"Yes, why?"

He leaned close and whispered, "Are you separating?"

"No. He's shopping for his parents."

This little incident became the highlight of our week as we chuckled over it. The humor gave us strength to go on. It was an amusing break from the unreality of our lives. Humor is a necessity, just like communication.

Look for ways to rejuvenate yourself and to enjoy the few remaining months or years your loved one has on this earth.

Chapter 9

Conclusion

As you gradually say goodbye to your parent or spouse, try to keep a positive attitude. Enjoy the moments that he or she is back in the real world and can say, "I love you." Cherish the smiles and the moments of laughter. If I'm not traveling I visit my mother once or twice a day, not out of guilt, but because I know she is losing her ability to communicate. Each moment we have in which we can still verbally interact is a blessing. Another reason I visit so often is for the first time since I left home, we live close to each other. It's fun to be able to take a walk and pop in for a few moments to see how she is doing. I also have the privilege of a flexible schedule. Any extra time I spend with Mom during the day can usually be made up with late nights at my computer.

Create special memories. Throw parties. Go on outings if possible. Your loved one may not remember the events, but you will. My brother is able to have long conversations with Mom by talking about the good old days; her memory of the younger years of her life is still strong.

It can be a favorable advantage to let others politely know what is happening to your family member. The first year Mom showed no interest in sending out Christmas cards I sent cards explaining Mom's disease. The outpouring of love she received from old friends calling or writing was amazing.

Get help from professional agencies like the Alzheimer's Association, the National Council on the Aging, and Catholic Community Services. Join a support group. It helps to talk to others as your loved one travels this difficult road. Accept help, and don't let guilt add extra stress.

It is hard to watch our loved ones gradually disappear. Hopefully the information in this booklet will make your journey easier.

• • •

I would like to add a personal note. There is only one way my husband and I have been able to keep going while caring for our parents; we turn to our Lord and Savior Jesus Christ. We pray for guidance and the ability to go on. We refresh ourselves in His Word. We know that we can do all things through Him who gives us strength, (Philippians 4:13).

If you do not have a personal relationship with Jesus Christ, I would like to invite you to enter into a relationship with Him. John 3:16 states, "For God so loved the world that He gave us His only begotten Son, that whosoever believes in Him should not perish, but have everlasting life." Simply believe that Jesus Christ died on the cross for your sins, and you will have eternal salvation. With that salvation you will enter into a relationship with Christ that will sustain you throughout this challenging journey.

I pray that you will find comfort as your loved one walks this path of a gradual disappearance.

Definitions

Merriam – *Webster's* definition of Alzheimer's:
A degenerative brain disease of unknown cause that is the most common form of dementia, that usually starts in late middle age or in old age, that results in progressive memory loss, impaired thinking, disorientation, and changes in personality and mood, and that is marked histologically by the degeneration of brain neurons especially in the cerebral cortex and by the presence of neurofibrillary tangles and plaques containing beta-amyloid — called also *Alzheimer's.*[4]

Alzheimer's Association's definition of Alzheimer's:
Alzheimer's disease is a progressive brain disorder that damages and eventually destroys brain cells, leading to loss of memory, thinking and other brain functions. Alzheimer's is not a part of normal aging, but results from a complex pattern of abnormal changes. It usually develops slowly and gradually gets worse as more brain cells wither and die. Ultimately, Alzheimer's is fatal, and currently, there is no cure.

Alzheimer's disease is the most common type of *dementia,* a general term used to describe various diseases and conditions that damage brain cells. Alzheimer's disease accounts for 50 to 80 percent of dementia cases. Other types include vascular dementia, mixed dementia, dementia with Lewy bodies and frontotemporal dementia.[5]

Mayo Clinic definition of dementia:
Dementia isn't a specific disease. Instead, dementia describes a group of symptoms affecting intellectual and social abilities severely enough to interfere with daily functioning. Many causes of dementia symptoms exist. Alzheimer's disease is the most common cause of a progressive dementia.

Memory loss generally occurs in dementia, but memory loss alone doesn't mean you have dementia. Dementia indicates problems with at least two brain functions, such as memory loss and impaired judgment or language. Dementia can make you confused and unable to remember people and names. You also may experience changes in personality and social behavior. However, some causes of dementia are treatable and even reversible.[6]

Merriam-Webster's definition of dementia: a usually progressive condition (as Alzheimer's disease) marked by deteriorated cognitive functioning often with emotional apathy.[7]

Suggested Resources

A Place for Mom
Catholic Community Services
HUD
National Council for the Aging
The Alzheimer's Association

Suggested Reading

The Emotional Survival Guide for Caregivers: Looking After Yourself and Your Family While Helping an Aging Parent by Barry J. Jacobs PsyD (Guilford, 2006) A compassionate book by an expert to help care-giving families avoid burnout.

The Circle by Sally Hughes Smith. Sally journals about the emotions she dealt with moving her mother out of her childhood home and into a memory care facility.

Still Alice by Lisa Genova. This book is written from the perspective of the patient dealing with early onset dementia.

Letters from Madelyn, Chronicles of a Caregiver by Elaine K. Sanchez. This book is a compilation of letters written by Elaine's mom to Elaine. It highlights the day-to-day challenges of being a caretaker.

Endnotes

1 *Wikipedia*, s.v. "Sundowning (dementia)," last modified December 12, 2011, http://en.wikipedia.org/wiki/Sundowning_(dementia).

2 Dr. Sameh Elsanadi, MD, Geriatric Psychiatrist, CEO of iCare Senior Solutions, LLC; quotes are provided for this booklet.

3 Dr. Joanne Marie Hamilton, PhD, ACPP-CN, Neuropsychologist, Director of Adult Neuropsychological Services Advanced Neurobehavioral Health of Southern California; quotes from Cognitive Factors Affecting Driving Safety Seminar conducted by Dr. Hamilton on July 13, 2011 at Aegis Living of Dana Point. Some information taken from TrafficSTATS.com developed by Carnegie Mellon Professors David Gerard and Paul S. Fischbeck

4 "Alzheimer's" (2012). In Merriam-Webster Dictionary Retrieved from www.merriam-webster.com/dictionary/Alzheimer's

5 "Alzheimer's" (2012). At Alzheimer's Association website. Retrieved from www.alz.org/research/science/alzheimers

6 "Dementia" (1998-2012). At Mayo Clinic website. Retrieved from www.mayoclinic.com/health/dementia

7 "Dementia" (2012). In Merriam-Webster Dictionary. Retrieved from www.merrian-webster.com/dictionary/dementia

A portion of the proceeds from the sale of this booklet will be donated to the Alzheimer's Association.

To find out more about Elizabeth Lonseth and her other publications please visit
elizabethlonsethnovels.com

31942002R00040